BEAT

THE USMLE

STEP 2 CS

James D. Lawrence III

Vinnie Leduc

Dedicated to our parents

Thank you so much for your unconditional love, undying support, and endless sacrifice. We love you dearly.

Amazon Creat Books

Cumming , GA 30040

Thank you very much for purchasing this review of the United States Medical Licensing Examination, Step 2 CS (Clinical Skills).

Compared to the other big daddy that may or may not be looming in the not-too-distant future (that would be Step 2 Clinical Knowledge, of course), Step 2 CS focuses on the techniques that you've integrated into your method of approaching the patient encounter… the skills, as the title of the exam suggests. "Well, obviously," you may be muttering to yourself. "What did I just buy?"

Oh, we'll tell you what. You've bought the single guide that will provide the boost you need for self-comforting confidence when you feel like you're about to lay a brick of you-know-what a few seconds before the very first encounter. You've bought the extra oomph that will help you leave this exhausting marathon with the peace of mind that you've nailed it, instead of second-guessing and torturing yourself for the next 1-4 months while you wait for your results.

We started this review by saying thank you, but by the end of this whole thing, we want you to be thanking yourself! So let's get on with it and BEAT Step 2 CS! Also, we'll refer to the test as just "CS" from here on out.

One of the smartest guys I know told me that CS was the hardest test he'd ever taken. We'll get back to that assertion later, but the point is:

DO NOT OVERLOOK STEP 2 CS.

If you're reading this guide, you're one step ahead of others and one step further from the cardinal sin of brushing CS off. We know plenty of people who made this crippling mistake, and we don't want you to do the same.

Most students pass this test. The numbers vary each year, but an overwhelming majority of students pass Step 2 CS. Do you want to be in the minority? Do you want to spend another $1,250 or $1,480 (plus any traveling/lodging expenses) and more time studying and preparing for this? The process of finding a test date that works for your schedule (if you're currently in rotations) and that releases your results out in time (if you're applying for residencies soon) is a long one that can be a huge headache!

Back in the day, this test used to be the ECFMG Clinical Skills Assessment. ECFMG stands for the Educational Commission for Foreign Medical Graduates, so it was basically designed to weed out foreign medical school students and graduates who didn't communicate well enough, including a-holes with horrible bedside manner. That's why sometimes when sought for advice on CS, older residents and attendings may dismissively say, "If you speak English, you'll be fine."

That may have been the case a few years ago, but just recently in 2013, the passing requirements for the exam were raised, particularly in the ICE (Integrated Clinical Encounter) category. This is the category that includes your very important note-writing, as opposed to the other two categories (Communication and Interpersonal Skills;

Spoken English Proficiency). By the way, if you fail one of the three categories (**ICE**, **CIE**, **SEP**), you fail the entire Step 2 CS. That means you can NOT pass this test simply by speaking English and being familiar with medical jargon like the way Leonardo DiCaprio's character was in *Catch Me If You Can* when he faked being a pediatrician. Do you concur?

This leads us back to the overview of the test, which is below and taken verbatim from the USMLE Step 2 CS website:

"Step 2 of the USMLE assesses the ability of examinees to apply medical knowledge, skills, and understanding of clinical science essential for the provision of patient care under supervision, and includes emphasis on health promotion and disease prevention. Step 2 ensures that due attention is devoted to the principles of clinical sciences and basic patient-centered skills that provide the foundation for the safe and effective practice of medicine.

Step 2 CS uses standardized patients to test medical students and graduates on their ability to gather information from patients, perform physical examinations, and communicate their findings to patients and colleagues."

Look at that. The word "knowledge" comes before "skills." This guide can't teach you all the medical knowledge you'll need to be a successful physician or even all the medical knowledge you'll need to pass this test. For that, we highly recommend the bible for Step 2 CS, aka **First Aid for the USMLE Step 2**. This guide is a great complement to, but by no means a replacement of, that wonderful and thorough book. If you for some reason don't have time to read that entire book, we recommend that you read as many of the longer practice cases in the second half of that book as you can, then go through the short section on difficult questions and their appropriate responses.

Although we can't magically transfer to you all the medical knowledge you'll need, we *will* underline and hit the key points that will be important and useful for your interviewing and note-writing. And like the overview stated above, we will also cover the exam's "emphasis on health promotion and disease prevention." Lastly, we will reinforce the "basic patient-centered skills" that aren't just important for this daylong test, but essential for your career as a doctor who cares.

Now let's get back to the interesting claim that CS was the hardest test my good friend had ever taken. There's definitely an argument for that, and that argument has to be rooted in the fact that CS is unlike most other exams.

While its overall length can be about an hour short of the grueling experience that is Step 1 or Step 2 CK, CS requires you to be on your feet. Literally. You'll need to be fully engaged and at the top of your game while you interact with standardized patients (SP).

Observing and catching their subtleties. Choosing what to ask and say. Deciding what to scribble down onto your notes. Selecting relevant parts of the physical exam. Actually performing them correctly. Answering any curveballs the SPs throw at you. All while developing a differential diagnosis.

That's over half of the time spent away from a computer. What little time you do spend at a computer will be filled with furious clacking away on the keyboard as you type up the note.

It's exhausting! CS is a mentally and physically taxing test. It's a marathon, except actual marathons take less time. But like a marathon, you should train for CS.

We're not just talking about the two days or two weeks you've set aside right before the test to get through those practice cases. We're also talking about the invaluable practice you'll get in your rotations. Practice makes perfect, right? Or as close to perfect as you can get.

You should already be interviewing real patients and writing notes during your clerkships. If not, volunteer to do so. If hospital protocol doesn't allow students to submit notes into the EMR, practice writing them on paper, or do them in your head at least. You want to do this as much as possible to get your brain accustomed to spitting out a template until it becomes second nature by the time you take CS, when

TIMING IS CRUCIAL.

The most common complaint by far that we've heard (and can attest to as well) is that there's not enough time. The most common denominator we've noticed from students who've admitted failing CS is that they ran out of time while writing the note for at least one patient.

Fifteen minutes is the maximum amount of time you'll get with the patient. If you leave the patient room before 15 minutes are up, you can use the precious extra few seconds or minutes on writing your note only, which you'll have at least 10 minutes for.

That makes a total of 25 minutes for each case. Almost half an hour sounds sufficient, but if you hesitate a couple times, don't know what you're doing, or don't have a system down, you'll wish each and every time that you really did have a full half hour.

That's why practice is so important in your preparation for CS. If your school offers mock CS exams, take advantage of them! You will not regret the extra time spent on not just getting past the shock of uncertainty during your first few cases, but also shaping your own methodical system.

Big events aren't much different. Sports have scrimmages, and shows have rehearsals. Is it a coincidence that timing is crucial in both? You can compare CS to a fancy game that you can beat. It's essentially an interactive show or carefully constructed simulation with highly trained actors as the patients. Well, you're an actor, too! And you've just spent the last several weeks or months immersed in clinical rotations, a great way to research the role!

Whatever way you want to look at it, get your head in the game and

PRACTICE.

Many students like going through the First Aid practice cases with a partner, and we recommend that. Time the interview and physical exam, too! Switch back and forth with a friend who's also going to take the exam. Ask your significant other to be the patient; this also works as another excuse to touch your beloved... just don't let any physical exam escalate into one of your fantasies on the actual test day! Okay, back to being semi-professional.

Practice your patient encounters with a clipboard, a couple sheets of paper, and two pens (what you'll get on exam day).

Practice typing your 10-minute notes here:

http://www.usmle.org/practice-materials/step-2-cs/patient-note-practice2.html

What you see in that link is very similar to what you'll see on the screen after every patient encounter.

We'll go over some specific note-writing tips later, but the point now is to practice until you have your own personalized system down. Speaking of which, that all starts with what you decide to do in

the first 20 seconds

of every patient case. You'll all be lined up in front of different doors. A voice on a loudspeaker will instruct the SPs to get ready. You might hear yours rustling about behind the door, but what should be on your mind?

Relax, and remember you know what's coming. Training for this pretty much started years ago when you entered med school. You've jumped through all the hoops so far, and you'll jump through this one toward earning that M.D. behind your name. Easily if you've been reading this.

Take a deep breath. Say a prayer. Close your eyes and meditate for a few seconds. Or stare at the little sliding compartment in front of you on the door.

"Examinees, you may begin."

Your 15 minutes with the SP officially starts now. Slide the little window thing over to reveal a sheet of paper with basic information and vitals on your upcoming patient.

Don't enter the room just yet; take 20 seconds or less to jot a few things down first.

Here are some suggestions on what to write before entering the room:

1. The last name of the patient: This is so that you can address the patient as "Mr./Ms./Mrs./Dr. [LAST NAME]" throughout the encounter.

2. The chief complaint of the patient: He or she will tell you this again once you're inside, but writing the CC down will get your noodle subconsciously started on forming a differential diagnosis. It may also help trigger additional questions or observations if you hit a wall and get stuck during the encounter.

3. Any abnormal vital signs: These are probably the least important things on this list, but they may also help trigger additional questions if you hit a wall.

4. Mnemonics to guide your interview: By test day, you should already have a good sense of what questions to ask in every scenario. However, writing down a mnemonic can also help if you get stuck. Consider writing OPQRSTAAA down vertically along the left side of your paper. In response to your first open-ended question, the patient may rattle off info that answers some of those, which you can quickly jot notes of next to the corresponding capital letter. Now make sure you ask the patient about the remaining letters of the mnemonic.

The patient info on the front door will be available to you again after the encounter while you write the note, so don't worry about mining it for every last details before you enter the room.

Once you have your pre-encounter notes ready, get ready to meet and greet the patient. Congratulations, you've completed the first 20 seconds like a champ. 24:40 to go! Then all over again 11 more times.

Knock on the door and wait for the SP to say, "Come in." Go in, close the door, and quickly confirm their identity. ("Ms. Connor?" "Yes.")

Introduce yourself properly and shake the patient's hand.

"Good morning, Ms. Connor. My name's Dr. Bauer, and I've been asked to see you regarding your [pain/leg/child/concern]. Before we get started, I want to assure you that everything here is strictly confidential, aside for a few exceptions that I'll let you know about if they come up. I'll ask you a few questions, maybe do a quick physical exam, and then we'll discuss my impressions and work together to get a better idea of what's going on. Is it all right with you if I take notes?"

You can score a bunch of points here with an intro like that. Also be sure to make good eye contact when you shake the patient's hand.

<u>Good morning, Ms. Connor</u>: You've greeted the patient, and by using the patient's surname, you've planted the seeds for a personal yet professional relationship. Don't use the patient's first name even though you'll have it from the info sheet outside. In your practice one day in the future, you can say, "Wassup, Sarah!" or whatever you like. But not here.

<u>My name's Dr. Bauer</u>: You can introduce yourself as a medical student, but you're allowed to call yourself a doctor here. Do it. It exudes confidence, which may help you subconsciously play into that role better and may help the SP (who is grading you for the next 14:40) subconsciously evaluate your performance more favorably.

<u>I've been asked to see you regarding your [pain/leg/child/concern]</u>: Incorporating the

chief complaint into your introduction will keep you in the right mindset, which is to continuously develop your differential diagnosis. Don't say "problem" because it may connote a stigma.

Before we get started, I want to assure you that everything here is strictly confidential: You can leave the rest of this part out if you feel like it's a mouthful. The important thing is that this bit about confidentiality hits something few students remember to include. Additionally, it further develops patient-physician trust and encourages the patient not to hold back on any potentially embarrassing or disturbing info.

I'll ask you a few questions, maybe do a quick physical exam, and then we'll discuss my impressions and work together to get a better idea of what's going on: Two big things here. Firstly, you're communicating to the patient what's about to go down. Adopt this habit for the rest of your encounter.

Secondly, by saying "we" and "work together", you are further building a relationship in which the patient is engaged and is at an equal level to you.

Is it all right with you if I take notes?: Also get into the habit of seeking permission. Remember to do so before asking "more personal questions" before exploring the social history, before beginning the physical exam, and before untying or moving the patient's gown.

Begin the interview with an open-ended statement.

For example, something like "Tell me about your cough" or "So what's the story with your arm?"

While you take notes, make sure you maintain as much eye contact as possible, and don't keep the clipboard in between the patient's face and yours. While writing, make confirmatory responses, such as nodding your head or repeating key words.

Do not forget to note any relevant observations about the patient, such as grimacing, crying, poor eye contact, speaking softly, restless foot tapping, and anything out of the ordinary. Not only will you report these in your typed note, but they may also be clues pointing at a diagnosis.

Round out the interview with OPQRSTAAA

Onset – When did this start to occur? What was the patient doing? Did it begin gradually or suddenly?

Progression – What has happened since the onset? Has it gotten any better or worse? Has the patient noticed any changes?

Quality of pain – How would the patient describe the pain? Sharp? Dull? Burning? Sore? Cramping? Tearing? Crushing? Throbbing?

Region/**R**adiation – Ask the patient to point to the specific location, and if relevant (e.g. pain or rash), find out whether the problem is moving.

Severity – Ask the patient to rate the pain on a scale from 1 to 10, and make sure you describe what each end of the spectrum signifies.

Timing – Has the patient ever experienced this before? If so, how often? Is it constant or intermittent?

Alleviating Factors – Does anything make it better or give the patient some relief?

Aggravating Factors – Does anything make it worse?

Associated Symptoms – Has the patient noticed anything else happening during this episode? This is a good way to catch some things that the patient may have forgotten, and it also can lead you to ask about other specific symptoms that may be related.

Anytime a patient complains about pain, say that you're sorry to hear about that, and ask if there's anything you can do to make the patient more comfortable.

If the patient coughs, offer a tissue and some water. If the patient sneezes, offer a tissue. If the patient hiccups, offer some water. If the patient burps or farts, consider further investigation only if it may be relevant to the chief complaint.

Always inquire about personal medical history because even "with no PMHx" will be at or near the beginning of the HPI for your note later. Don't forget about family history.

Ask the patient if it's okay to ask "more personal questions about your lifestyle" before jumping into the social history.

When you're done, summarize the key positive and negative findings. Then, ask if there's anything else the patient would like to add or may have forgotten to mention.

Certain cases will require further investigation that's more focused and tailored to the scenario.

If the SP admits to any type of **bodily fluid or discharge** (vomit, diarrhea, urine, nasal, vaginal, wound, nipple, etc.), consider the following simple set of questions.

Amount & **A**roma? – Ask for an estimate.

Blood? – This is the most important one!

Color & **C**onsistency? – Color is usually more important. If you forget to ask about consistency (slimy/runny/grainy/etc.), then the patient will hopefully tell you this when you ask for any other ways to

Describe it, please.

If the patient is female and has a complaint related to her womanly parts, you'll have a lot of more things to explore.

Make sure you make a note to yourself to mention in your discussion later that a pelvic exam must be done in the future.

Vaginal Symptoms: Itching? Burning? Discharge? Spotting? Odor? Cramping?

Menstruation: Last Menstrual Period? Regularity of periods? Length of periods? Age of menarche? Tampons/Pads? (How many daily and over the course of the period?)

Sexual History: Currently Active? How many partners now and in the past? Contraceptive use? STDs or STIs?

OB History: Pregnancies? Abortions? Miscarriages?

PAP smear: Date of last PAP smear? Results?

If she has **irregular menses**, ask about the following:

Anorexia/**A**ppetite

Brittle **B**ones

Coronary Artery Disease / **C**hest pain

Dryness between the thighness (vagina)

Eating/**E**xercise habits

Flashes (Hot Flashes)

If you have a patient with abnormal bruising and seems reluctant to answer your questions, then you may have an **abuse victim**.

Tell the patient, "I want to remind you that I'm bound by law to keep everything here strictly confidential, and I'm my main concern is to be here for you and to help you."

Proceed with **SAFEGUARDS**

Safe: "Do you feel safe at home?"

Alcohol & drugs: "Does he abuse alcohol or drugs?"

Family & **F**riends: "Is anybody else aware of what's going on?"

Emergency Plan: "Do you have an emergency plan?"

Guns & Weapons: "Are there any guns or other weapons at home? Has he ever threatened you with one?"

Unwanted Sex: "Does he force you to have sex with him?"

Absent/**A**fraid: "Is he here now? Are you afraid he'll be home later?"

Relationship: "How is your relationship with him?"

Depression: "How have your appetite and sleep been?"

Suicide: "Have you ever thought of ending it all yourself?"

Go through **SIGECAPS** if you suspect depression:

S – Sleep disturbance (increase/decrease)? Ask: "How has your sleeping been lately?" (Response: "I sleep all the time and don't feel like getting up, doc.")

I – Interest loss? Ask: "What do you do for fun?" (Response: "I used to watch plenty of movies, but I haven't felt like it recently.")

G – Guilt / Hopelessness / Worthlessness / Regret? Ask: "Do you feel guilty or remorseful?" (Response: "I don't know... I do feel worthless and like a waste of life.")

E – Energy decrease? Ask: "How would you describe your energy level recently?" (Response: "Little to none. I don't know what's wrong with me.")

C – Concentration decrease? Ask: "Any difficulty concentrating?" (Response: "I'm sorry, what'd you say?" Actually, it'll be more like, "I think so.")

A – Appetite change (increase/decrease)? Ask: "How has your appetite been?" (Response: "Honestly, I don't ever feel like eating.")

P – Psychomotor retardation or agitation? Technically, you will have likely already observed that the SP has been moving very slowly in general, but to be complete with this popular mnemonic and to show the SP that you know what you're doing, take a few seconds to ask, "Have you noticed anything different in regards to your movement?" (Response: "...Um... I think so...")

S – Suicidal Ideation? Ask: "Any thoughts of suicide?" (Response: "Sometimes I do want to end it all...")

Make sure you conclude this set of questions by thanking the patient for sharing their answers. This is also another opportunity to reinforce your relationship with the patient.

(Example: "Ms. Downer, thank you very much for opening up to me. I realize that telling me all of this is difficult, but it will help us get to the bottom of this together so that you can get the best help possible.")

Be mindful that you are still being evaluated on empathy, so don't rush through these questions too quickly, or you may be docked points for seeming to be too insensitive. On the other hand, you're on a time crunch, so don't linger either. If the patient remains quiet and hasn't answered your question after a few seconds, then say, "I know this is tough, Ms. Downer. Is there anything I can do to make you feel more comfortable?" Offer a tissue if you haven't already, then move on to the next question.

Because **diabetes type 2** continues to be a huge and growing problem, be prepared to have a diabetic patient by remembering to cover the following topics and to likely counsel on them if necessary.

medications and compliance

glucose and HbA1C (routine monitoring? last measurement?)

lifestyle (diet, exercise, sex)

eyes (changes in vision? routine visits to optometrist?)

recurrent infections and slow-healing wounds

extremities (numbness? tingling? routine visits to podiatrist?)

recognition & treatment of hypoglycemic episodes (from overmedication)

If you have a **male patient with urinary complaints**, don't forget to mention the need for a rectal exam to examine the prostate during the discussion at the end of the encounter, and make sure you go through

FINISHED PUBS

Frequency

Incontinence

Nocturia

Incomplete emptying of bladder

Smoking & **S**exual history

HEsitancy & **HE**maturia

Dribbling & **D**rugs

Pain & **P**yuria

Urgency

Burning

Straining & **S**tream power

Another common complaint that you'll definitely encounter as a future physician is **joint pain or arthritis**. That means there's a good chance that you'll get an SP that presents with this. Make sure you go through

CITRUS

Color change (bruising) & **C**rackles

Infection recently? (for Reiter's)

Tick bite? **T**rauma? **T**emperature around joint?

Rash & **R**edness

Urinary symptoms? (for Reiter's)

Swelling & **S**tiffness

Here's a good mnemonic for a chief complaint of jaundice:

JAUNDICE BITS

Joint pain

Abdominal pain

Urine & stool color

Nausea & vomiting

Diarrhea

Itchiness

Constipation

Eating habits, appetite/weight change

Blood transfusion in the past

Immunization history

Temperature (fever) & **T**ravel

Sexual history

WHAT TO DO WHEN YOU DON'T KNOW WHAT TO DO

First of all, relax. Take a second to take a deep breath and remind yourself that you've prepared sufficiently for this test, especially if you're reading this guide. You know your stuff.

The CS brain fart happens to almost everyone. Realize that some cases will be either quite vague or similar to one another or both. Every case isn't meant to have a single straightforward diagnosis.

The main point of CS is to evaluate whether you behave appropriately and investigate appropriately. It's about your method, and this includes how you handle brain farts.

Without any lifelines, **remain calm and confident**.

If you have no clues or leads during your history taking after asking everything you can think of, the following question can do wonders:

"What do *you* think could be the cause of all this?"

For example, (and this is a true story,) I had a middle-aged woman who complained of blood in her stool, but all of her answers to my questions were negative and gave me absolutely nothing to work with.

So I asked her, "What do you think might have caused this?" And she replied, "Well, last night I had anal sex with my husband for the first time."

Eureka! Bingo! Ding, ding, ding! That basically gave me everything I needed for the rest of the encounter.

We've gotten reports of some patient actors who will be helpful and give you little hints (wink, wink) or subtly guide you. They might cough, even straight-up blurt out something they hadn't before, or repeat something before that you didn't focus on.

These SP actors aren't here to make your life miserable and aren't here to fail you, even in a case that's meant to incorporate a difficult or uncomfortable situation, such as an impatient, confrontational, or distrustful SP.

This is why it's important that you start every encounter pleasantly and show from the very beginning that you really care about what's going on and that you're not doing things robotically or just going through the motions.

If you show them this and they see that maybe one day you'll be the kind of doctor that they would want to have themselves, then they're more likely to help you out with unsolicited hints.

Another thing to consider doing when stuck is to quickly **summarize everything**, including the positives and negatives, that the patient has told you. That way maybe it will trigger your memory to something you may have overlooked, or maybe even trigger the SP's memory.

Some information that SPs give is actually designed to not come out the first time you asked, so it's okay to ask again. Usually these responses are ones that are more psychological or relate to abuse, depression, or embarrassment.

They may take some coaxing, and this is not unlike the real-life encounters where patients tend to hide stuff they don't want to tell their doctors until you've earned their trust.

It pays to be nice and to show empathy. Anytime somebody reveals information that is even mildly embarrassing or private or difficult for them to give, I always tell them that I appreciate them sharing that information with me.

If you've gone through the history taking and still don't know what to do, then move onto

the physical exam

and stick to the following strategy, which should be the way you tackle every physical exam (PE):

Do the most relevant test(s) first, then round out the rest of the physical exam with shortened versions of the Basic 3 (we'll go over that soon). If the most relevant test is already one of the Basic 3, then just complete the other two parts.

Remember that your physical exam should start about 7-8 minutes into the encounter. If the loudspeaker announces the 5-minute warning, then finish the interview ASAP (like in the next 15 seconds) and ask the patient if you may do a short physical exam.

Before you begin the PE, you have the option of either washing your hands or putting on gloves. Since proper handwashing is supposed to take two sing-throughs of the "Happy Birthday" song (about 15 seconds), we suggest slapping on some gloves instead. So try out which size is most comfortable and easiest for you to put on while you're in the orientation/break room before the test starts.

In the 5-10 seconds it should take you put on gloves, you can use this time to ask any questions you may have forgotten. If you've got nothing else, then now's the time for quick chitchat with the SP.

If a holiday is coming up, ask about any special plans. Ask specific questions about how work or school is going. Comment on *something*, preferably something the SP can relate to.

This keeps your communication with the SP, an important part of your CS evaluation, flowing while avoiding an awkward silence as well.

Before each and every part of the PE, you should ask for permission to proceed. After you've completed each part, thank the patient.

You don't need to explain your findings during the PE (or ever, unless the SP specifically asks), but sandwiching each part of the PE with permission and thanks should be firmly integrated into your technique.

At the very minimum, your PE should include

The Basic 3

We're not going to teach you every detail of each part of the PE because you should know these things by now, but we will emphasis some key points.

1. Basic Pulmonary Exam: Ask for permission to undo the patient's gown from the back. Warm up the stethoscope with the palm of your hand (important!), and instruct the SP to take a deep breath in and out every

time the SP feels the diaphragm (say "stethoscope" though) placed on the SP's back. Don't rush through this part; allow the diaphragm to remain on the SP's back for the full breath before moving on to the next spot on the back. Make sure none of those spots are over either scapula! You can go through the motions here, but don't be sloppy! And... that's it for the basic pulmonary exam! Surprised?

Now this is just the bare minimum of this part of the PE. If you think your SP's complaint calls for it, then you better do the rest of the pulmonary exam, including palpating, tactile fremitus, vocal fremitus, and whispered pectoriloquy. Before you move on to the next part of the Basic 3, don't forget to thank the patient and ask for permission to proceed to...

2. Basic Heart Exam: This is pretty similar to the Basic Pulmonary Exam. Ask the patient if you can lower the gown from the front, and warm the stethoscope up again. Start at the appropriate place for the aortic valve, then pulmonary valve, tricuspid valve, and finally mitral valve. Spend at least a couple seconds listening to each spot, and check for the point of maximal impulse. That's it! Like with the previous part, if the patient's complaint is cardiovascular-related or warrants a full cardiac exam, then you sure as hell better do that. Once this is done, tie the SP's gown up from the back (doesn't have to be a crazy knot) before moving on to the last part of the Basic 3:

3. Basic Abdominal Exam: As always, thank the patient for allowing you to complete the previous part of the PE, and ask for permission to proceed to

this part. Then ask the patient to lie down, and make sure you pull the leg tray out (familiarize yourself with the exam center's bed during orientation). Ask for permission to move the patient's gown up just enough to expose the abdomen. Warm the stethoscope up once again, and gently lay the diaphragm in all four quadrants for a couple seconds each. Once this is done, tell the patient, "I'm going to press lightly onto your tummy, so just tell me if there's any pain at all, okay?" Throughout your light palpation, look at the patient's face to check for any grimacing. Now tell the patient, "I'm going to do the same thing but press a little harder now. Please let me know if there's any pain, and I'll ease up. Is that okay?" Again, watch the SP's face during deep palpation. Once that's done, you're done with the Basic Abdominal Exam!

Remember that if relevant, you should check for Murphy's sign, psoas sign, obturator sign, Rovsing's sign, and all that good stuff. We're not Bates, but we recommend you refer to Bates for complete instructions on each PE technique.

This is one last reminder: the Basic 3 parts of the PE are the bare minimum! Do not neglect to perform the set of tests that is most relevant to your patient's complaint FIRST, *then* round out your PE with the Basic 3 if you have time.

Your entire, focused PE should take about 5-6 minutes. Timing is crucial, remember? So practice your technique and have your method down cold!

The Discussion

By the end of your interview and physical exam, you should have about 1-2 minutes to wrap up your patient encounter.

It's definitely fine not to reveal to the patient a definitive diagnosis at this time. If you don't know, be honest and tell the SP that "at this time, there's a variety of things that can explain your symptoms."

Inform the patient, "I want to do some simple tests that can help give us a better idea of what's happening." Here's where you include the no-no tests that you couldn't perform today, like the breast exam, pelvic exam, and rectal exam. Just don't forget to mention these if they're relevant!

Don't go into medical mumbo-jumbo. Say "blood test", not "CBC". X-rays are fine, but if you mention CT scan, don't give the patient an opportunity to ask what that is exactly. Say, "We'll do a CT scan, which is just like an

X-ray, except a little fancier and shows us more of your body like slices in a loaf of bread." Do the hand motion like you're slicing up some yummy bread. "Don't worry; it's totally painless."

If there's any counseling to do, now is also the time to do it. This could be about diabetes, smoking, drug abuse, unprotected sex, and other dangerous lifestyle elements.

Do not be condescending or patronizing. Maintain courtesy and focus on the fact that you're here for the patient and can offer whatever help the patient seeks.

Wrap up the discussion by asking, "Do you have any other concerns or questions for me?" The patient may indeed bring up a difficult or random question here. If you don't remember the appropriate same responses from First Aid, just answer with tact and calmness. Be politically correct and sensitive, and you will be okay.

Now the patient encounter is really ending. If there's nothing else to address, thank the patient one last time, shake the patient's hand while making eye contact, and give the patient a goodbye that he or she will remember.

For example, do a callback to a previous comment you might have made while putting on your gloves. Refer to an upcoming holiday that may be right around the corner. Something like "Have a safe Fourth of July, Mr. Dumphy" or "Have a wonderful Thanksgiving, Mr. Lannister."

At the very least, tell the patient to take care and have a great week or weekend.

The Patient Note

Once you've exited the patient room, there's no going back. You now have 10 minutes plus whatever extra time you may have gained from leaving the patient encounter early to whip up a patient note.

We must emphasize again that practicing the note is very important, so here's that link again:

http://www.usmle.org/practice-materials/step-2-cs/patient-note-practice2.html

Use it! Before you regurgitate all your history findings, type the first line of the history as "XX-year-old male/female with PMHx of XXX presents with CC."

Then, transfer all of your history notes onto the next 14 lines of the history window. If examinees were given more time, we'd write the HPI in paragraph form like most normal people. But since you don't have much time, you'll find it easier to write the HPI in bullet form. Don't forget to include the family history and social history, too.

You can save a lot of time in the next window, the physical examination, by practicing and spitting out a basic template. Start with a general line that includes a simple description of the patient (obese, anxious, well-nourished, etc.) that also mentions whether the patient was alert and cooperative and whether the patient was in any acute distress.

Now it's time to rattle off negative results that you should have memorized:

Lungs: Clear to auscultation bilaterally; no rubs, wheezes, or rhonchi.

Heart: RRR; S1 and S2 heard with no murmurs, rubs, or gallops

Abdomen: ND, NT to palpation, bowel sounds heard, no guarding or rebound tenderness

Remember that these patients are actors, so most of your physical exam will be negative. However, simulated findings, scars, and discolorations should all be recorded.

Adjust the template above accordingly to the actual results from your physical exam, then add the results of any additional tests you performed.

Now order your top 3 diagnoses. If you only have one or two, then that's fine.

Here's where you can save a lot more time, too. If you've learned the PC keyboard shortcuts for copying and pasting, you can just highlight lines from your HPI or PE, press Ctrl + C to copy them, then press Ctrl + V to paste them in the lines following each diagnosis that they support!

This is why practicing typing on that USMLE link is important!

Finally, list the diagnostic studies at the bottom of the page (including the no-no tests). Since students tend to run out of time with the patient note, this section at the end of the note is sometimes left blank, which is a HUGE mistake! Those are essential points, so you may consider filling those in first at the beginning of the 10 minutes in case you do run out of time.

One last thing: Stop when the proctors tell you. Don't you dare try to squeeze in a few more words. Doing so is like playing with fire... except your hands are already soaked in oil. You might get away with it, but if you're caught, you may get off the first time with a stern warning (if you're lucky). Otherwise, you'll be ejected. This isn't baseball. ONE or TWO strikes, and you're out! Just don't risk it. Besides, if you follow all of our advice here, chances are you'll be finishing in time.

When the twelve and final note is over, you're done! Don't think about what you might have forgotten or what you could have done. You passed if you followed this guide after going through First Aid! Congratulations, and go treat yourself to something nice!